DIY Healing Salve:

25 Amazing Homemade Recipes of Herbal Balms and Salves

Table of content

Introduction

Many of you must think that technology is the ultimate miracle throughout the history of mankind. No doubt technology has been an important element which has added utility in almost all walks of life. Its various dimensions are undoubtedly enhancing the effectiveness and efficiency. But technology can never stand as a replacement for natural remedies and natural solutions. In fact just as the human generation is moving away from nature there has been an increased rate of body ailments and other issues. Nature lies as the lifeline for all sorts of human life aspects so you can find a proper solution and guidance from the various creations of nature.

Just looking around the corners of nature you will find various botanical species and herbs which may look ordinary and tiny but provide a lot of utility and effectiveness related to various different aspects of human body and human health. Various different forms of herbal mixtures have been a part of human civilization for a long time and even today they stand as a good way of handling various issues of human health and vitality. Another group of herbal mixtures which are highly useful includes herbal salves and balms. These appear as one of the best remedies for a number of body maintenance and ailment issues.

Chapter 1 – Tips to Make Herbal Salves and Balm

No matter how much progress technology makes, the utility and usefulness of natural solutions can never be denied. It is because nature's creations are all based on the best principals, as the creator is always well aware of all the needs of the creations. Same has been the case for humans where all his needs can be best served by natural recipes and solutions.

Within the environment, you can see millions of different creations which can be used by human civilizations from fulfilling different needs. Not only the nutritional needs can be served by the natural resources but various other remedial purposes are also well served by the species present all around us.

Among the useful creations of nature, the herbal species and various plants forms cover a wide range of utilities which can be served best if these plants and herbs are explored well. Just as more and more wisdom is added to the stream of knowledge, explorations are taking place to make the best use out of natural remedies provided by nature. One such newer trend is that of herbal salves and balms which have added a revolutionary aspect in various domains of healing and recovery.

How do Herbal Salves work?

Herbal salves are a modification made to use the medicinal herbs and botanical species in such a way that their effectiveness and healing power is enhanced. Herbal salves are combinations of herbs along with some organic oil. It allows the herbs to get infused in the concentrated oils to end up in a concentrated and wholesome form of herbal salves. The organic oil provides the deep and quick penetration ability to the salves whereas the herbs bring along various soothing and healing properties.

What purpose they can serve?

So together these two ingredients make up the best combination for providing treatments of various different skin and body issues like:

- Stress relief

- Sore muscles

- Skin irritations

- Minor cuts

- Minor burns

- Itching

- Insect bites

- Chest congestion

Making herbal balms and salves at home:

One of the best things about herbal salves which enhance the utility is the ease of making them at home. Because of fewer ingredients used and easy availability of the equipment you can easily make a wide range of these herbal balms and salves at home.

Just like another homemade recipe which you follow for cooking, you also need to follow some recipe for this balm and salves. Along with that, you must keep in mind some quick tips which will surely ease the process of making these balms. These tips belong to general process followed for making balm and salves and do not relate to some specific recipe only:

- If you want to follow the best process and you want your herbal balm to be effective it is advisable to use mason jars. These canning jars are best for preparation and storage of oils and herbs.

- The quality of essential oil being used is highly critical. It is advisable to use virgin oil so that the real content and extract of oil remains present in your herbal balm.

- For the effective preservation of herbal balm, it is essential to follow a thorough and effective strain process. Any of the foreign particles present in your jar can affect the utility and storage life of your herbal balm and salve so it is essential to follow a careful process.

- One of the tips to heat up the herbs having a lot of moisture is to cook them in an uncovered pan. In this way, the moisture present in the herbs will get heated quickly and the time duration to make the herbal salve will greatly reduce.

- While selecting any of the herbs make sure that you are picking it up from a valid and authentic store. Buy natural and fresh herbs so that the real purpose of making herbal balm can be ensured.

- Once you are done with the process of making these balms it is highly advisable to keep them safe. Excessive light and heat can reduce or even eliminate the healing properties of balms so keep them in air tight jars.

Chapter 2 – Recipe to Make All-purpose Salves

The herbal balms have the capacity to serve a number of different purposes. From healing to relief, these salves and balms have the potential to serve you the best. Below are some recipes to make these herbal miracles at home.

1. *The soothing salve*

Ingredients:

- Beeswax Base

- Coconut Oil- 1 c

- Olive Oil (extra virgin)- 1 c

- Beeswax – 2 tbsp

- Vitamin E capsules- 2

Directions:

Arrange an accurately sized double boiler for making this salve. Put the boiler on the stove and make sure that you keep the flame to a medium intensity. You do not need to boil up the water. The boiler is just heated enough so that all the ingredients get thoroughly mixed after getting mild heat. Now first of all pour olive oil. In next step pour coconut oil. Continually move the spatula to avoid lumps of coconut oil. When you see a uniform consistency of the oils, add beeswax and stir continually. Now use some piercing equipment to puncture the capsules for getting vitamin E. turn off the heat and add vitamin E. mix well and store the salve in some airtight jar or bottle.

2. Skin soothing salve

Ingredients:

- Clove Oil- 3 drops

- Frankincense Oil - 6 drops

- Lavender Oil- 6 drops

- Rosemary Oil- 6 drops

Directions:

Get hold of an accurately sized double boiler for making this salve. Put the boiler on the stove and make sure that you keep the flame to a medium intensity. You do not need to boil up the water. The boiler is just heated enough so that all the ingredients get thoroughly mixed after getting mild heat. Now first of all pour clove oil. It will have a strong smell. So it is better to add it first. Now add rest of oils one by one and keep stirring. This natural salve will help in soothing your skin and for making your skin even and rupture free.

3. All-purpose coconut salve

Ingredients:

- Coconut Oil- 1/4 c

- Cocoa Butter - 1/4 c

- Shea Butter - 1/4 c

- Almond Oil - 1/4 c

- Vitamin E capsules - 2

Directions:

Get hold of an accurately sized double boiler for making this salve. Put the boiler on the stove and make sure that you keep the flame to a medium intensity. You do not need to boil up the water. The boiler is just heated enough so that all the ingredients get thoroughly mixed after getting mild heat. First of all, add cocoa butter so that it will serve as the base of the salve. Wait for two minutes so that it gets evenly dispersed. Now add both of the oils followed by Shea butter. You will need to stir these ingredients continually. After turning off the heat, add vitamin E by rupturing the capsules with some clean needle. Transfer in a glass jar.

4. *Coconut and Patchouli salve*

Ingredients:

- Chamomile Oil- 8 drops

- Myrrh Oil - 8 drops

- Patchouli Oil- 2 drops

- Lavender Oil- 4 drops

- Cocoa Butter - 1/4 c

Directions:

First of all, heat up a boiler, at medium heat intensity. It will serve as a good mixing area for all of the ingredients. Although cocoa butter may take the time to melt yet you do not need to burn it out. Put boiler over the flame and add cocoa butter first. Once you are sure that cocoa butter is melted properly add up all of the oils one by one and stir well. Pour in some air tight jar.

5. *Geranium salve*

Ingredients:

- Beeswax- 3 tbsp

- Geranium Oil - 3 drops
- Lavender Oil- 6 drops
- Rosemary Oil - 6 drops

Directions:

Get hold of an accurately sized double boiler for making this salve. Put the boiler on the stove and make sure that you keep the flame to a medium intensity. You do not need to boil up the water. The boiler is just heated enough so that all the ingredients get thoroughly mixed after getting mild heat. Add beeswax first so that it may serve as a good base for all of the essential oils. Now add oils one by one and make sure that you do not allow them to get cooled down during the process. When you start smelling the oils turn off the heat and transfer the salve to some air tight jar.

6. Shea butter salve

Ingredients:

- Shea butter – ½ cup

- Chamomile oil - 8 drops

- Myrrh oil - 8 drops

- Rosemary oil - 6 drops

- Patchouli oil - 2 drops

- Lavender oil - 4 drops

Directions:

For this recipe of all-purpose balm, you will have to get an accurately sized double boiler for making this salve. Put the boiler on the stove and make sure that you keep the flame to a medium intensity. You do not need to boil up the water. The boiler is just heated enough so that all the ingredients get thoroughly mixed after getting mild heat. Shea butter will serve as the base of this salve so it must be melted prior to adding oils. Add it in the boiler and wait till it gets evenly mixed. Now add oils one by one and mix well followed by storage of salve in some air tight jar.

7. *Rosemary salve*

Ingredients:

- Coconut Oil - 1/4 c

- Cocoa Butter - 1/4 c

- Shea Butter - 1/4 c

- Rosemary Oil - 1/4 c

- Vitamin E - 2 capsules

- Myrrh oil- 2 drops

Ingredients:

This combination of rosemary oil with cocoa butter base will serve as one of the best combinations for making an all-purpose salve. Get hold of an accurately sized double boiler for making this salve. Put the boiler on the stove and make sure that you keep the flame to a medium intensity. You do not need to boil up the water. The boiler is just heated enough so that all the ingredients get thoroughly mixed after getting mild heat. Add the base first so that it gets melted enough. Now add oils and butter. Heat till get melted. After turning off the heat, add up vitamin E.

Chapter 3 – Recipes of Herbal Balms for Pain and Headache

In our day to day lives sudden pains, especially headache, may cause serious unrest. Rather than using some chemical based medicine you can use the herbal balms specially made for pain relief. Some of the recipes for these pain relief balms are mentioned below:

8. Peppermint Headache balm

Ingredients:

- Peppermint oil – 10 drops

- Lavender oil – 8 drops

- Beeswax- 2 tbsp

Directions:

We have mentioned the ratio of beeswax and oil for a normal balm. If you want to change the consistency you can add it as per your choice. Adding more oil will result in an even creamier balm. However, adding more beeswax will result in a solid balm.

Mix together beeswax and oil in a saucepan. You can also use a metal bowl to serve the purpose of the double broiler. If you are quite interested in making herbal balms and salves at home, it is recommended to fix one pan for this purpose. Heat up the wax and once it turns into a liquid add up the oils. Peppermint has a strong refining effect. Pour into a container and wait till the salve gets cooled down. Let it harden and then apply using small pieces.

9. *Burn balm*

Ingredients:

- Calendula Flowers - 1 part

- Comfrey Leaves - 1 part

- Comfrey Root - 1 part

- Hypericum perforatum Flowers

- Olive Oil – 2 parts

- Beeswax (grated) – 1 part

Directions:

Place the calendula flowers along with comfrey roots and leaves over the upper portion of the double boiler. Also, add olive oil. Oil will also be added in the upper portion of the boiler. The lower part of the boiler will be filled with water. Do not overheat the water. Just bring it to the low boil.

Allow the oil to simmer mildly for around 30minutes. However keep an eye on the oil and checking after regular intervals so that oil may not get overheated. After heating the oil use a strainer to shift it to a small pan. Now add beeswax. Now heat the mixture again so that the wax gets evenly mixed with oils. Although you will get a good consistency of balm with these ingredients but you can also check the appropriate consistency of balm by placing it into the freezer. Add more oil or wax as per your need. Stir the balm properly in glass containers.

10. *Cuticle healing balm*

Ingredients:

• Coconut oil - 1 tbsp

• Almond oil - 1 tbsp

• Hemp oil - 1 tbsp

• Mango butter - 1 tbsp

• Beeswax (grated) - 1½ tbsp

• Lavender oil-10 drops

• Peppermint oil - 5 drops

• Eucalyptus oil - 5 drops

• Fennel oil - 5 drops

• Clary sage oil - 5 drops

Directions:

Use a double boiler in order to melt the oils, mango butter and beeswax. When all of these ingredients get evenly melted and mixed, turn off the heat. Now add oils one by one and stir with the spatula. Transfer to pot and wait till the balm fixes. Apply a label so that the balm can be used by everyone at home, in the case of need.

11.Foot pain balm

Ingredients:

- Pure lanolin - 4 oz.

- Raw beeswax - 1 oz.

- Olive oil (with infused calendula flowers) - 1.5 oz.

- Shea butter - .5 oz.

- Cocoa butter - .25 oz.

- Neem oil - 1/2 teaspoon

- sea buckthorn oil - 1/4 teaspoon

- vitamin E oil - 1ml

- lavender oil - 1ml

- rosemary essential oil - 1ml

- fir needle oil - 1ml

- tea tree oil - 1ml

- rosemary extract - 1ml

Directions:

This mixture of ingredients can turn into miraculous relief balm for foot pain. Mix together beeswax and oil in a saucepan. You can also use a metal bowl to serve the purpose of a double broiler. If you are quite interested in making herbal balms and salves at home, it is recommended to fix one pan for this purpose. Heat up the wax and once it turns into a liquid add up the oils. Pour into a container and wait till the salve gets cooled down. Let it harden and then apply using small pieces.

12. Jojoba headache balm

Ingredients:

- Chamomile dried herbs- 5 oz.

- Jojoba oil

- Beeswax – 2 tbsp

- Peppermint oil – 10 drops

Directions:

You will need to infuse the oils 3 weeks using a securely sealed container. Make sure to avoid any growth of the mold. If seen, you will need to start the process again. After the infusion period, use the strainer to separate out the herbs. Take a saucepan to mix wax and oil over a very low flame. Now pour in some glass container and let it get harder at room temperature.

13. Pain soothing balm

Ingredients:

- Olive oil – 2 tbsp

- Chamomile oil - 8 drops

- Myrrh oil - 8 drops

- Rosemary oil - 6 drops

- Shea butter – 2 tbsp

Directions:

Add up Shea butter in a boiler but make sure to give it a very mild heat. When the wax gets melted, add the oils one by one and stir well. Now transfer in glass jars having the tight lid. The balm will get hardened at room temperature.

Chapter 4 – Lip Balms to Make Your Lips Beautiful

14. Almond lip Balm

Ingredients:

- Beeswax – 1 oz.

- Cocoa Butter – ½ oz.

- Essential Oil - 1 oz.

- Sweet Almond Oil

Directions:

First of all Melt, Cocoa Butter, Beeswax and Almond Oil by putting in the microwave. Use the Defrost Power option, applying intervals of 1 minute to blend. When entirely melted, mix essential oil like Spearmint oil. You can also use any oil in citrus flavor. Combine carefully. Cautiously pour into jars or tubes. Let the balm cool down completely. This recipe can make up to 12 tubes.

15. Balm for glossy lips

Ingredients:

- Coconut Oil (Extra Virgin) – 1 oz.

- Vitamin E Oil - 1.5 tbsp

- Beeswax (Cosmetic Grade) - 2 oz.

- Vanilla oil - 25 drops

- Colored lipstick – ½ inch slice

Directions:

First of all melt Beeswax and coconut Oil by putting in the microwave. Use the Defrost Power option, applying intervals of 1 minute to blend. When entirely melted, mix Vanilla oil and Vitamin E oil. Combine carefully. Now when you see that all ingredients are well mixed put the slice of colored lipstick into the mixture. Store continuously. It will add a shine and color to your balm but this step is optional. If you want transparent balm you can skip this step. Cautiously pour into jars or tubes. Let the balm cool down completely.

16. Healing balm

Ingredients:

- Coconut oil- 1/8 c

- Vitamin e oil - 1/8 tbsp

- Shea butter - 1/2 tbsp

- Cocoa butter -   1/2 tbsp

- Honey - 1/2 tbsp

- Cocoa powder - 1 tbsp

- Peppermint oil - 3 drops

- Beeswax

Directions:

Put the cocoa butter and Shea butter in a double boiler. Also, add coconut oil. Now turn on the boiler at an over VERY low intensity for around 20 minutes, stir intermittently. Make sure that the temperature of the mixture does not go above 175 degrees. Now mix beeswax and stir again. When you can see melted beeswax, turn off the heat of boiler and pour essential oil and Vitamin E oil. Whisk well while mixing oils. Check for any kind of lumps present in the balm. Transfer to an airtight glass container.

17. Moisturizing balm

Ingredients:

- Grated beeswax - 1 1/2 tbsp

- Shea butter - 1 1/2 tbsp

- Jojoba oil - 1/2 tbsp

- Almond oil (sweet) - 1/2 tbsp

- Sweet orange oil – 4 drops

- Vitamin e oil - 10 drops

Directions:

Melt Shea butter, beeswax, and oils collected in a big double boiler. When thoroughly, melted turn off the heat. Wait till the beeswax mixture gets cooled down. But do not wait till the wax gets fixed again. Now start adding orange oil along with Vitamin E and almond oil. Mix and decant into balm containers. Wait till the balm gets solidified. The balm must be hard enough to be used as a lip balm. If you are not satisfied with the consistency of balm you can always add wax or oil in it to make the consistency as per your need.

18. Healing lip balm

Ingredients:

- Almond oil- 1 cup

- Echinacea root - 1 teaspoon

- Comfrey leaf - 1 teaspoon

- Plantain leaf - 1 teaspoon

- Calendula flowers - 1 teaspoon

- Yarrow flowers - 1 teaspoon

- Rosemary leaf - 1 teaspoon

Directions:

You will need to infuse the oils 3 weeks using a securely sealed container. Make sure to avoid any growth of the mold. If seen, you will need to start the process again. After the infusion period, use the strainer to separate out the herbs. Take a saucepan to mix wax and oil over a very low flame. Now pour in some glass container and let it get harder at room temperature.

19. Pink lips balm

Ingredients:

- Grapefruit seed extract – 2 tbsp

- peppermint oil – 10 drops

- grated Carrot – ¼ cup

- Olive Oil – 4 tbsp

- Almond Oil (Sweet)- 4 Tbsp

- Honey - 2 Tbsp

Directions:

Heat up the almond oil and olive oil in a small saucepan. Make sure to keep the intensity of the flame very low. Now gently add carrots into the mixture of oil. Cover up the pan by placing a lid. Let it simmer for around 20 minutes on low flame. Stir occasionally. Now remove from heat. Now let the mixture remain at room temperature so that the carrots get infused in oil properly. After the prescribed time use the strainer to pour oil in a separate jar. Mix honey and stir well. In order to use this balm dip a cotton bud in the pan and ten apply over the lips to get shiny pink lips.

Chapter 5 – Herbal Salve and Balms for Pet Animals

Herbal salves are surely one of the greatest remedial content available for our use. But to your surprise, these salves and balms are not only useful for human body and its various ailments but these are multipurpose elements which can also be used for a variety of purposes. One such use of herbal salves is to apply it for your pets. Below are some most useful herbal salve recipes which you can follow for your pets.

20. Animal salve

Ingredients:

- Coconut Oil – 1/2 cup

- Olive Oil – 1/2 cup

- Beeswax – 1/4 Cup

- Melaleuca oil – 15 drops

- Lavender oil – 15 drops

- Peppermint oil –10 drops

Directions:

First of all melt the olive oil, coconut oil, and beeswax by pouring all of these in a medium saucepan. Make sure to keep the heat to a medium intensity. When all of the three ingredients get thoroughly mixed, it is now time to turn off the heat remove the pan. Let the pan stay at room temperature for almost 15 minutes. Now start adding oils one by one. During the pouring, the process makes sure that you stir the mixture evenly so that any kind of lumps may not form. When you see that the mixture has shifted to an evenly thick balm, transfer it into a glass container.

21. Pet warming balm

Ingredients:

- Coconut oil - 1 cup

- Olive oil - 1 cup

- Beeswax pastilles - 4 tablespoons

- Lavender oil - 12 drops

- Frankincense oil - 12 drops

- Pepper oil - 40 drops

- Vitamin e oil - 1/2 teaspoon

Directions:

Firstly add up olive oil, coconut oil, and beeswax in Mason jar with a wide mouth. Now place this glass jar in a pan containing simmering water. Stir infrequently till the wax get properly melted and all of the other ingredients are fully combined. Now pour the oils into the jar. Now pour melted oils within the jars oolong with the essential oils. Fill up the jar with oils leaving a space of around ¼ inch from the lid. Now place a paper towel and let the ingredients cool down at room temperature for 8 hours. Do not place the lid during these 8 hours of cooling. Once properly made and cooled down you can save this balm up to six months.

22. Herbal salve for dogs

Ingredients:

- Sunflower oil- 2 oz.

- Almond oil (sweet) – 2 oz.

- Coconut oil – 2 oz.

- Shea butter – 1 oz.

- Beeswax – 4 tbsp

Directions:

Get hold of an accurately sized double boiler for making this salve. Put the boiler on the stove and make sure that you keep the flame to a medium intensity. You do not need to boil up the water. The boiler is just heated enough so that all the ingredients get thoroughly mixed after getting mild heat. First of all, add Shea butter so that it will serve as the base of the salve. Wait for two minutes so that it gets evenly dispersed. Now add all the oils one by one followed by Shea butter. You will need to stir these ingredients continually. Transfer in a glass jar.

23. Bug repellent balm

Ingredients:

- Coconut oil - 1/4 cup

- Shea butter - 1/8 cup

- Beeswax granules - 4 tsp.

- Citronella oil - 12 drops

- Rosemary oil- 8 drops

- Cedarwood oil - 8 drops

- Calendula flowers – a handful

- Lemongrass oil - 8 drops

- Eucalyptus oil- 8 drops

- Tea tree oil - 8 drops

Directions:

Place the calendula flowers over the upper portion of the double boiler. Also, add Citronella oil. Oil will also be added in the upper portion of the boiler. The lower part of the boiler will be filled with water. Do not overheat the water. Just bring it to the low boil. After five minutes add rest of the oils and allow the oil to simmer mildly for around 30minutes. However keep an eye on the oil and checking after regular intervals so that oil may not get overheated. After heating the oil use a strainer to shift it to a small pan. Now add beeswax. Now heat the mixture again so that the wax gets evenly mixed with oils. Although you will get a good consistency of balm with these ingredients but you can also check the appropriate consistency of balm by placing it into the freezer. Add more oil or wax as per your need. Stir the balm properly in glass containers.

24. Dog paw balm

Ingredients:

- Olive oil – 2 oz.

- Sunflower oil- 2 oz.

- Almond oil – 2 oz.

- Tea tree oil – 2 oz.

- coconut oil – 3 tbsp

- Shea butter – 1 oz.

- beeswax – 4 tbsp

Directions:

Arrange an accurately sized double boiler for making this salve. Put the boiler on the stove and make sure that you keep the flame to a medium intensity. You do not need to boil up the water. The boiler is just heated enough so that all the ingredients get thoroughly mixed after getting mild heat. Now first of all pour olive oil. In next step pour coconut oil. Continually move the spatula to avoid lumping of coconut oil. When you see a uniform consistency of the oils, add beeswax and stir continually. You can change the consistency of the balm if you find it too hard by adding some more sunflower oil and heating it well. Once you are satisfied with the consistency of the balm store the salve in some airtight jar or bottle.

25. Herbal salve for cats

Ingredients:

- Rose oil - 5 drops

- Lavender oil - 4 drops

- Ylang Ylang oil – 3 drops

- Shea butter – 2 tbsp

Directions:

Add up Shea butter in a boiler but make sure to give it a very mild heat. When the butter gets melted, add the oils one by one and stir well. Now transfer in glass jars having a tight lid. The balm will get tough at room temperature.

Conclusion

Just as the human civilization has moved away from nature's principles, the quality of life has been affected. The technology was added to the human life to enhance ease and utility but because of its uncontrolled and poorly managed use, the aftermaths of this excessive use have been drastic. So we can see a lot of different health and social issue emerging in the new generations. The best solution for sorting any problem of human life and body still lies in the use of nature's solution because these solutions are based on the wisdom and intellect which is far better and sophisticated than the technology-based solutions.

A lot of medical and national research is being carried out in today's scientific world where a lot of chemicals are added to food and medicine so that any problem of the human body can be healed. But as far as the comparative utility and effectiveness are concerned the natural solutions still appear to be the best. These solutions do not extend any kind of side effect so the effectiveness is high. One such example is that of the extended focus being put forward to the use of herbal balms and salves. These combinations of oils and herbs appear to cater a lot many human body issues without any kind of side effects. This book has provided the simplest recipes for these balms so that people can easily follow the procedures at home. Just as you will explore more about these natural herbs and oils you will be able to make the even greater variety of salves.

FREE Bonus Reminder

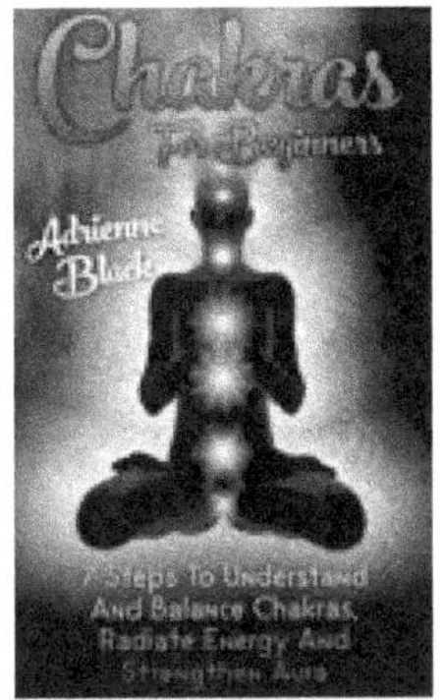

If you have not grabbed it yet, please go ahead and download your special bonus E book *"Chakras for Beginners. 7 Steps To Understand And Balance Chakras, Radiate Energy, And Strengthen Aura"*.

Simply Click the Button Below

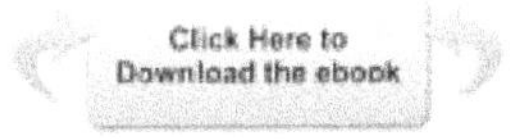

OR Go to This Page

http://lifehacksworld.com/free

BONUS #2: More Free & Discounted Books & Products

Do you want to receive more Free/Discounted Books or Products?

We have a mailing list where we send out our new Books or Products when they go free or with a discount on Amazon. Click on the link below to sign up for Free & Discount Book & Product Promotions.

=> Sign Up for Free & Discount Book & Product Promotions <=

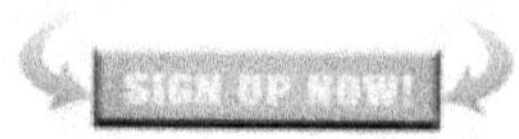

OR Go to this URL

http://zbit.ly/1WBb1Ek